MW01268718

DBT WORKBOOK

FOR KIDS

A FUN-FILLED JOURNEY WITH RONNY THE FRENCHIE TO LEARN
MINDFULNESS, BUILD SOCIAL SKILLS, REGULATE EMOTIONS, AND TACKLE STRESS

Table of Contents

ricca_garden

info@riccagarden.com

Published & Designed in

Brisbane, Australia

First print: Oct 2024

© Ricca's Garden. All rights reserved. No part of this publication may be reproduced, distributed, or transmitted, in any form or by any means, including photocopying, recording, or other electronic or mechanical methods, without prior written permission of the publisher, except in the case of brief quotations embodied in critical review and certain other non-commercial uses permitted by copyright law.

Disclaimer Notice:
Please note the information contained within this document is for educational and entertainment purposes only. All effort has been executed to present accurate, up to date, reliable, complete information. No warranties of any kind are declared or implied. Readers acknowledge that the author is not engaged in the rendering of legal, financial, medical or professional advice. The content within this book has been derived from various sources. Please consult a licensed professional before attempting any techniques outlined in this book. By reading this document, the reader agrees that under no circumstances is the author responsible for any losses, direct or indirect, that are incurred as a result of the use of the information contained within this document, including, but not limited to, errors, omissions, or inaccuracies.

A Note to Kids

Hi Kids! It's me, Ronny the Frenchie. I'm a fun-loving, curious canine, here to join you on your next big adventure! I love exploring and learning new things, especially when I can share the experience with friends like you.

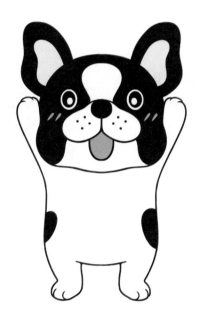

Just like humans, I have a bunch of different emotions. You can usually tell how I am feeling by looking at my body. If I'm hanging my head with my tail between my legs, I am probably scared or ashamed. When I feel angry or threatened, I growl and bare my teeth. Most of the time, these emotions pass quickly, but sometimes, I get overwhelmed and need some help.

Can you remember a time when your emotions overwhelmed you? When this happens, it's difficult to think about or do anything else, so it can really get in the way of school, friendships, sleep, and other activities.

Luckily, there are ways of managing your emotions so they are not so overwhelming. One of those ways is DBT.

What is DBT?

DBT stands for Dialectical Behavior Therapy and it's a kind of therapy for people who struggle with emotions, including anxiety, depression, anger, and shame. DBT teaches you ways of coping with these difficult feelings so they don't get in the way of your life, relationships, or happiness.

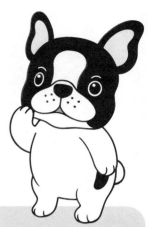

DBT has four main parts

Mindfulness

Mindfulness means being fully focused on the present moment instead of getting distracted by thoughts of the past or worries about the future. Mindfulness helps you become more aware of your thoughts, feelings, and urges so you can handle them better.

Emotion regulation

Emotion regulation is about understanding your feelings and learning how to manage them so they don't overwhelm you. By learning about emotions and how they are connected to thoughts and behaviors, you can lessen their effect and feel better more often.

Distress tolerance

Distress tolerance helps you cope with negative emotions so that you don't accidentally make the problem worse. It helps you see that thoughts and feelings don't last forever and there are things you can do to make it through even the most difficult situations.

Interpersonal effectiveness

Interpersonal effectiveness helps you be more successful in your relationships. This includes getting what you want out of talking to someone, building and keeping friendships, and feeling good about yourself.

Part 1
Mindfulness

What is mindfulness?

Have you ever been sitting in class but instead of focusing on what your teacher is saying, you are thinking about something your friend said the day before? Or at sports practice, you miss your coach's instructions because you are worrying about the next game.

When the mind gets bored or stressed, it often wanders to thoughts of the past or worries about the future. Mindfulness helps you stay focused on your current experience.

Have you ever tried to do homework while watching your favorite movie? Texted one friend while trying to hold a conversation with another? Even if you are really good at multitasking, something gets lost when you try to do too many things at a time. The homework has more mistakes, the movie is less enjoyable, and both friends can tell that you are distracted.

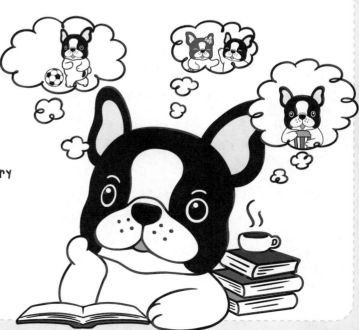

Mindfulness means doing one thing at a time and fully participating in that activity.

It has two parts: awareness of what you are doing in the present moment and acceptance of your thoughts, feelings, and sensations without judgment.

The second piece is harder than it sounds! I can't tell you how many times I have been on a walk with my human but instead of enjoying the experience, I'm fixated on some small annoyance like an itch under my collar. Mindfulness has taught me to accept the unpleasant parts of my experience and observe my urges without immediately responding to them. Do you know what happens to an urge when you don't respond to it? It often goes away!

Mindfulness has tons of other benefits, too.

It reduces stress, anxiety, and depression and improves sleep. It makes you more aware of yourself, helps you cope with physical illness, and may even help you get better grades in school! Here are a few other ways mindfulness can help you:

Control of mind

Mindfulness directs your attention to the task at hand so you don't get caught up in negative thoughts like past mistakes or worries about the future.

Control of emotions

Mindfulness helps you understand your feelings and manage them better so that they are less overwhelming.

Control of behavior

Mindfulness helps you pause and think about how you want to respond to a challenging situation.

Improved memory and concentration

Mindfulness helps you focus, making it easier to remember important information.

Activity 1

How Mindful Are You?

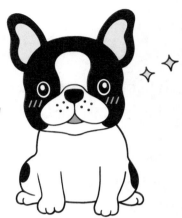

If you've ever used a map to try to get from point A to point B, you know that in order to get where you want to be, you have to know where you are. This activity is all about figuring out where you are, mindfulness-wise. Hopefully, after answering the following questions, you'll have a better sense of your strengths and areas for improvement.

Unlike the tests you take in school, this test has no wrong answers and no grades! So be as honest as possible because this activity is just for you.

How often do you have the following experiences? Answer "always," "sometimes," or "never."

1. When you're going somewhere, you feel like you're acting automatically, moving without paying attention, maybe not even remembering how you got there.

        Always   Sometimes   Never

2. When you spend time with your family or friends, you find yourself thinking about other things instead of being fully present with them.

        Always   Sometimes   Never

3. You have a lot of worries or thoughts about the past or future.

        Always   Sometimes   Never

4. You find it difficult to focus on one task or activity without getting distracted.

        Always   Sometimes   Never

5. When you're doing something fun, you catch yourself thinking about something else instead of enjoying the moment.

        Always   Sometimes   Never

6. You try to do more than one thing at the same time, like eating while watching TV or doing homework while chatting with a friend.

Always   Sometimes   Never

7. You feel disconnected from your surroundings or the people around you.

Always   Sometimes   Never

8. When you're doing your homework, you get distracted by thoughts about something else instead of focusing on your work.

Always   Sometimes   Never

9. You say or do something without thinking, like yelling at someone or taking part in risky behavior.

Always   Sometimes   Never

Looking back on your answers, in what situations are you the most mindful? When do you find it the most challenging to stay mindful? How could mindfulness help you personally? Write your answers below:

I am most mindful when _____

I find it challenging to be mindful when _____

Three ways that mindfulness could help me are:

1. _____

2. _____

3. _____

Activity 2
Getting Back to Your Senses

Self-discovery can be unsettling. When I took the "How Mindful Are You?" test, I was shocked to discover how often I get distracted! But then I decided to use it as an opportunity to learn and grow. I made plenty of mistakes in my quest to become more mindful, but I also learned a lot! And now I get to guide you on the same journey.

In this activity, we'll use the 5 senses to practice being mindful. We'll focus on one sense at a time, starting with sight. You can do this activity while walking in nature, enjoying a meal, taking a shower or bath, or even waiting in line.

Ready to try it?

 First, use your eyes to slowly look around at your surroundings. Notice any shapes, patterns, colors, and movements. Make sure to look up, down, and behind you as well as to each side. Choose one object and examine it more closely, noting what makes it unique.

 Now, move on to your ears. Listen for hard-to-hear sounds like the wind in the trees as well as loud ones like city traffic. Which sounds are sharp or high-pitched? Which are soft and soothing? Are the sounds continuous or do they come and go? Is there any rhythm to the sounds?

 Next, use your nose to identify any smells in the area. Is someone cooking nearby? Can you tell what spices or other ingredients they are using? What does your nose tell you about the plants in the area—any flowers or fragrant trees? What man-made scents can you identify?

 Now, tune into your sense of taste. Take a small bite of food and hold it in your mouth. Notice how the food tastes and feels. Is there any change in temperature or texture as the food mixes with saliva? Pay attention to how these things change as you chew. Finally, swallow slowly and mindfully, focusing on how the food feels as it moves down your throat.

Finally, what can you touch? If you are sitting, notice the sensation of your legs on the chair and your feet on the ground. Where do your clothes contact your skin? Do they feel rough or smooth? How does the air feel—warm or cold, still or breezy?

Use this table to record your observations:

Activity	
Sights	
Sounds	
Smells	
Tastes	
Feelings	

Which parts of this activity were the most challenging?

Was there anything you found surprising?

How can you use your 5 senses to be more mindful in your everyday life?

Activity 3
No Time Like the Present

We dogs are really good at staying in the present. Whether chewing a bone or enjoying some belly rubs, we are usually focused on the here and now.

Human brains are built differently from dog brains, so staying in the present might be harder for you than it is for me. Not to worry! In this activity, I'm going to teach you how to focus on the task at hand and let go of any distractions.

Ready to get started?

Choose something you do regularly, like brushing your teeth or taking a shower. The next time you do it, try focusing 100% on that activity. If you notice your mind wandering, try to observe this without judgment. For example, my mind often wanders to thoughts about food. Whenever I find myself dreaming about my next meal, I just say to myself, "Silly Ronny, you're missing what's happening right now!" Then, I gently direct my mind back to my present activity.

One thing that might help with this is to imagine you are training a puppy. When I first moved in with my humans, I had to learn when and where I could do my doggy "business." At first, it was really hard. I would get excited and forget to go where I was supposed to!

Luckily, my humans were very patient with me, never yelling or calling me names. This helped me learn that if I had to "go to the bathroom," as you humans say, I had to alert the humans to take me outside.

In this activity, when your mind wanders to something other than the present, imagine you are gently guiding a puppy back to the task at hand.

Use the log on the next page to keep track of your mindfulness activities!

Mindfulness Tracking Sheet

Date	What I did mindfully	Length of practice	What I noticed (thoughts, emotions)
Example: 24/07/20xx	Brushed my teeth	2 minutes	Emotions: Worried Thoughts: I was thinking about a test I have coming up. I gently reminded myself to focus on the brushing and enjoying the smell of the minty toothpaste.

Activity 4

A Breath of Fresh Air

If you're like me, you probably don't think much about your breath. There are just too many more exciting things to focus on, like squeaky toys! But the breath deserves some attention because it's kind of a mindfulness superpower. Mindful breathing activates your body's natural relaxation response, helping you to feel more relaxed and less stressed.

How do you breathe mindfully, you ask?

Well, I'm going to show you in this activity! The great thing about mindful breathing is that you can do it anytime, anywhere. Ready to get started?

Find a comfortable position, either seated with both feet on the ground, standing, or lying down. Now, bring your attention to the breath going in and out of your body. You don't need to try and control it in any way; just let it follow its natural rhythm and observe the following:

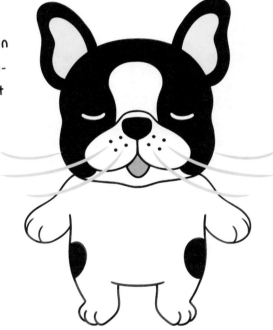

- Your belly rising as you breathe in and falling as you breathe out

- Your chest expanding as your lungs fill with air and then contracting as your lungs empty

- The brief pauses at the end of each breath in and breath out

- The feeling of the air as it goes in and out of your nose

If your mind gets distracted by some other thought or sensation, don't worry! Remember you are training a puppy, and gently guide your attention back to your breath.

You can also practice mindful breathing while walking.

First, use your footsteps to measure the length of your breath. I walk pretty fast (especially when I am on my way to my favorite dog park!), so I normally get 5 footsteps for each breath in and 4 for each breath out. You may get more or less—there is no "right" pace!

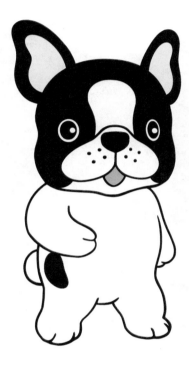

Now, try lengthening your breathing out by one step. What happens to your breathing in when you do this? Does it get longer or stay the same?

If it's comfortable, lengthen your breath out by one more step. Continue for 20 breaths, then breathe like you normally do.

Now, try this activity in reverse by slowing down your steps to match your breath—one step for each breath in, one for each breath out. This might feel awkward at first, but it's a great way to strengthen your mindfulness superpower!

Activity 5
Urge Surfing

There is something so soothing about watching the waves at the beach—don't you think? Each wave follows the same pattern, getting bigger and bigger until it crashes on the shore.

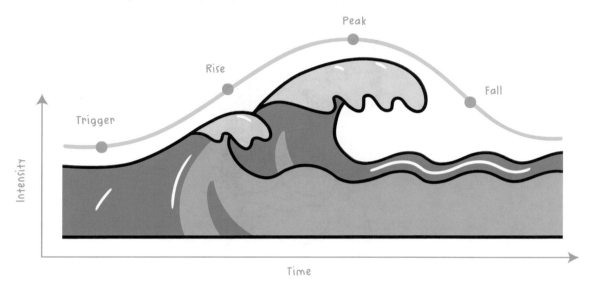

Urges follow the same pattern, starting small, becoming stronger, and eventually fading away.

You've probably experienced urges before. An urge is a feeling inside your body that makes you want to do something right away. Urges can be healthy, like when you have the urge to drink water when you are thirsty. But urges can also lead you to do things that are not good for you, like eating a whole bag of candy. Acting on these urges can cause problems in the long term. That's why it's important to be aware of your urges and learn to resist them.

In this activity, we are going to practice a skill called "urge surfing." Just like a surfer rides a wave to the shore, you are going to learn how to surf your urges as they rise and fall in intensity. This way, you can control your body instead of letting your urges control you!

First, think about what causes your urges. For me, it's usually the scent of some delicious human food. Before I know it, I'm jumping up on the table to steal my owner's dinner! Note that urges don't have to be about taking action. Sometimes, the urge can be to avoid someone or something (like my weekly bath—I always hide under the bed!)

What is an urge you've experienced recently?

Are there certain urges that are harder for you to resist? What are they?

The next time you experience an urge, imagine the urge is a surfboard and you are a surfer. Scan your body and notice any sensations connected to the urge. Where do you feel the urge the most strongly?

Can you use mindfulness to accept the urge and the discomfort that comes from resisting it? Or, is there something you can do to take your mind off the urge?

Just like actual surfing, you may not be successful your first time around. That's okay!

Keep trying, and each time you do it, you might find that you can "stay on the board" a little longer.

Activity 6
Thought Labeling

Have you ever watched the clouds go by, calling out shapes as you see them? (Personally, I see a lot of clouds that look like dog bones, but maybe that's a case of wishful thinking!) Clouds shift and change as they float in and out of eyesight. Even the largest and darkest clouds eventually move on, leaving clear skies behind them.

Your thoughts are like clouds. They come and go, gradually changing in shape and intensity. In this activity, we will practice letting our thoughts drift in and out of our minds like clouds in the sky. The goal is not to focus on any one thought but simply to notice it, label it, and let it go.

You have around 60,000 thoughts per day, but don't worry—we're not going to label all of them! In fact, most thoughts tend to be one of the following types: judging, worrying, planning, or remembering. You can also label your thoughts by the emotion you are feeling—"an angry thought," for example.

Let's have a go at this exercise:

1. Find a place where you are unlikely to be distracted and get into a comfortable position.

2. Close your eyes and take a few deep breaths.

3. Imagine your mind is a river and your thoughts are boats. You are sitting on the river bank, observing the boats (your thoughts) gently drift past.

4. Label each boat for the thought or feeling it represents. For example, the thought "Will I do well on my test?" would be a "worry boat." Try not to let any one boat carry you away—use your breath as an "anchor" that you can come back to as each boat passes.

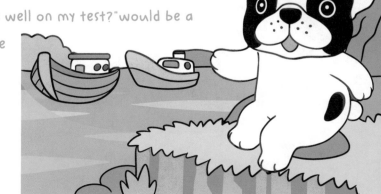

Ready? Set a timer for 2 minutes and write down as many thoughts as you can.

My thoughts	Label (e.g., "Worry Boat", "Happy Boat", etc.)

Reflection:

What did you notice? Were there a lot of boats with the same label?

Which boats were hardest to let go?

Choose a judgmental thought and rewrite it to fit the facts of the situation.

For example, I often have the thought, "I should be less hyper." My rewrite could be: "I have a lot of energy, so sometimes it's hard for my humans to keep up with me." If you get stuck, you can always try adding the phrase "I am having the thought that…" before your thought.

My Judgmental Thought:

Rewritten Thought:

How did it feel to rewrite your thought this way? Does it feel less factual?

Negative thoughts can make us feel stressed out or upset, but guess what? They're just thoughts, not facts! Learning to see them this way helps to remove some of their power. By being curious about our thoughts instead of judging them, we can be kinder to ourselves and others.

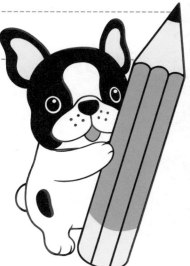

Activity 7

Focusing on the Good

Think back to the thought labeling activity on the previous page. How many of your thoughts were negative versus positive? Were the negative thoughts harder to let "float" down the river?

Sometimes, negative thoughts can get stuck, like boats on a sandbar, while the positive ones pass right through! But don't worry—I'm going to teach you how to hold onto the good boats with something called gratitude.

Gratitude means feeling thankful for things in your life.

These can be big things like friends and family or small things like the smell of cookies baking (mmmm… cookies!) Scientists have found that the simple act of listing what you're grateful for can help you feel better. Over time, it can increase the number of positive thoughts and make them more likely to "stick!"

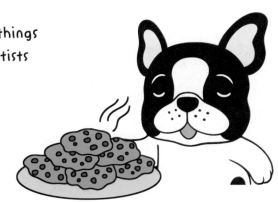

Ready to try it?

1. Think back on your day. List three things that went well or made you feel grateful:

----

2. If you like drawing, draw a picture representing what you are grateful for. Use colors and designs that make you feel happy.

3. If drawing isn't your thing, try writing a letter to someone about the good things that happened today.

As you draw or write, take a moment to really think about each happy thing.

How did it feel to focus on the positive? Were you surprised by the things that came to mind? I find that even on my worst days (getting shots at the vet!), I am able to find something to be grateful for (the nice lady who gave me the treat afterward).

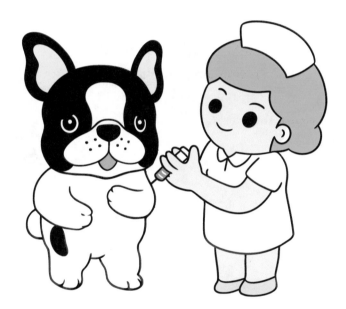

The goal of this activity is not to ignore or downplay the challenges in your life but to understand that what you focus on affects how you feel. When you think about what's going well and give thanks for the good things in your life, you feel happier.

Try doing this activity every night before bed, and before you know it, your river will be flooded with good boats!

Activity 8
Love Makes the World Go Round

So far, you've practiced being mindful of your senses, the present moment, your breath, urges, and thoughts. In this activity, we will use mindfulness to encourage two of life's most rewarding experiences: love and compassion!

Nothing is better than curling up next to my human and feeling their love—often in the form of belly rubs! And when my human is in pain or having a bad day, I make sure to give them extra kisses and cuddles to show them how much I love them.

Take a minute to think about the people you love.

Where do you feel this love in your body? For me, it is a warm and fuzzy sensation that starts in my belly and goes up to the tips of my ears!

Now imagine someone you love is suffering. How does this feel? While it might be less pleasant than the warm and fuzzies, compassion is a form of human connection. Compassion means sharing someone else's pain and helping them to feel better. Want to know something cool? When you show compassion to someone else, you often end up feeling better yourself!

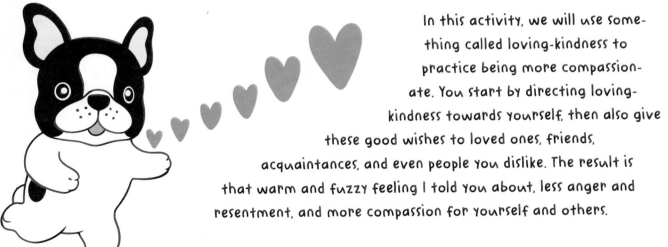

In this activity, we will use something called loving-kindness to practice being more compassionate. You start by directing loving-kindness towards yourself, then also give these good wishes to loved ones, friends, acquaintances, and even people you dislike. The result is that warm and fuzzy feeling I told you about, less anger and resentment, and more compassion for yourself and others.

Ready to get started?

23

Get into a comfortable position, either sitting, standing, or lying down. Open your palms to the sky, take a few deep breaths, and slowly repeat the following phrases:

May I be happy. May I be at peace. May I be healthy. May I be safe.

Focus on the meaning of each of these phrases. What would it mean for you to be happy, healthy, safe, and at peace?

After several minutes, give these wishes to someone you dearly love by replacing "I" with your loved one's name. Then, move on to someone who you neither like nor dislike—for example, someone you see regularly but do not know well. Next, see if you can give loving-kindness to an enemy or someone you find difficult to be around. Finally, direct the phrases towards all living beings:

May all living beings be happy. May all living beings be at peace. May all living beings be healthy. May all living beings be safe.

Reflection:

How do you feel after completing this activity?

Which parts were the hardest?

How can you use loving-kindness in your everyday life?

Activity 9
Accessing Your Wise Mind

When it comes to wisdom, owls get all of the credit. Sure, they have big eyes and heads that rotate 270 degrees, but that doesn't mean owls are the only wise animals in the world! You've got wisdom, too. In mindfulness, we call it "wise mind."

Wise mind is actually a mix of two different types of thinking: reasoning and emotional.

You use reasoning when you think logically about a problem and its solutions, using facts rather than feelings. Emotional thinking, on the other hand, is controlled by whatever you are feeling at the moment. You tend to lose sight of reason, facts, and logic when you are thinking emotionally.

Can you think of a time when you used each type of thinking? How did each situation turn out?

Wise mind uses a combination of reasoning, emotions, and intuition.

Intuition is that sense of knowing without a clear understanding of how you know. It's a "gut instinct" that guides you in challenging situations.

When you are in wise mind, you feel your emotions but are still able to think straight. You consider the pros and cons of different courses of action and make decisions that are best for you in the long run.

To better understand wise mind, imagine you are snorkeling in a cove. The water is clear and calm, so you can see straight to the bottom. You see shells, sea creatures, and kelp gently swaying with the current. Suddenly, a jet ski whizzes by, kicking up sand from the ocean floor. Your vision is clouded, and you lose sight of which way is up or down. You must wait until the sand resettles before deciding which way to swim.

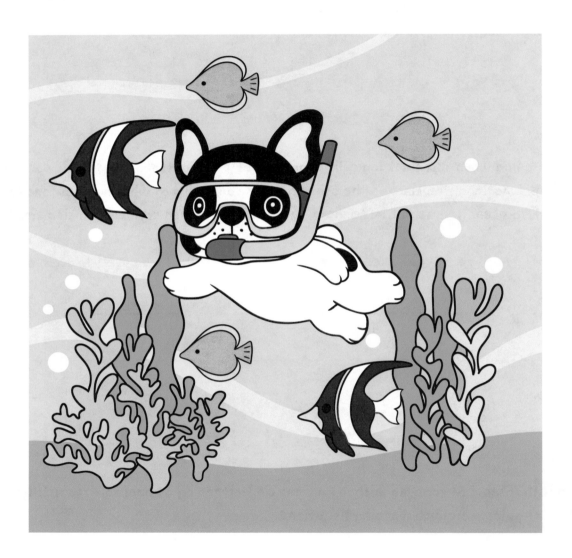

Emotion mind is like the jet ski, stirring everything up so you can't see the facts of the situation. Wise mind waits for the emotions to settle, then uses facts and feelings to decide what to do next. Mindfulness allows the water to clear so you can use wise mind.

The next time you experience a challenging situation, use one of the mindfulness activities in this book to find your wise mind and then ask it the following questions. Breathe in as you ask the question, then listen for the answer as you breathe out. Try not to actively search for an answer. Instead, just see what comes to mind.

- What is the right thing for me to do in this situation?
- What is the best way to handle how I feel right now?
- If I act on my emotions, what will the consequences be?
- What are the facts of the situation, and how can I use them to make a good decision?
- What are my strengths, and how can I use them to overcome challenges?
- How can I show kindness and compassion to myself and others right now?
- Is there a way to solve this problem that uses reasoning, emotions, and intuition?

How does wise mind feel different from emotion mind?

How can you use wise mind to manage your emotions and make better decisions?

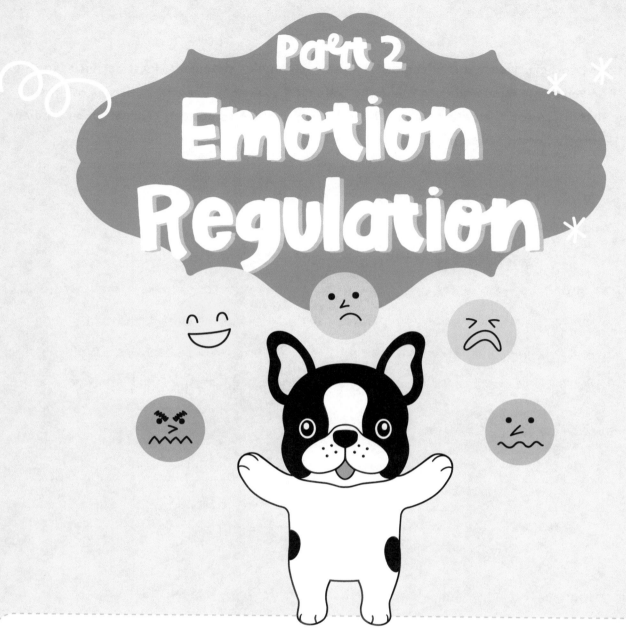

Part 2
Emotion Regulation

Congratulations! You have finished the first part of this workbook. How do you feel—excited, proud, skillful? Were there moments of frustration or discouragement along the way? How did you handle them?

In this part of the workbook, we will learn how to identify and regulate emotions, from joy to frustration and everything in between. Emotions are more than how you feel; they are also made up of thoughts, images, memories, and impulses. They can even lead to changes in your body, such as a faster heartbeat, sweating, and shortness of breath. Because emotions are so complex, the same emotion might feel different based on what's happening around you.

I used to think my emotions were a nuisance. I thought life would be so much easier if I didn't quiver in fear every time a big truck rumbled down the street or bark angrily at the mail carrier every time they tried to deliver the mail. But now I realize that emotions play an important role in our daily lives. Here are just a few things emotions do for us:

Motivation

Emotions prepare you for action! For example, fear helps you to run away from danger or stand up and fight to protect yourself. Emotions also help you overcome obstacles. Can you think of a time when you really wanted to win a game or do well on a test? That feeling helped you try your best, right?

Information

Emotions provide information about what is and is not working for you. For example, anger might tell you that someone is treating you unfairly. Guilt can be a sign that you have done something against your values. In this way, emotions can act as a kind of early warning system, appearing before your brain can fully process the situation. But sometimes, emotions can trick us into thinking something is true when it's not. Can you think of a time when you felt something was true that turned out to be false?

Communication

Emotions help you communicate. Think of a face-to-face conversation you had recently. How much did you understand from the other person's words, and how much from their facial expressions, body language, and tone of voice? These nonverbal signs help you know how others are feeling and vice versa.

Activity 10
Sentiment Self-Reflection

Remember the "How Mindful Are You?" test in Part I? This activity is similar, but this time, we are going to explore your emotions.

While we are all born with the ability to experience emotions, we must learn how to identify, express, and control them. Have you ever seen a toddler throw a tantrum? Toddlers are still learning how to effectively communicate and manage their emotions. But here's a little secret: toddlers aren't the only ones who experience emotional "meltdowns." We generally get better at managing our emotions as we get older, but none of us is perfect. Stress, hunger, or even just having a rough day can make our emotions trickier to handle.

Not to worry! We are going to learn a variety of skills to help you avoid emotional meltdown.

But first, let's take a few minutes to reflect on your current emotional experiences. As in the previous section, there are no wrong answers, so answer freely and honestly!

1. Do you feel comfortable discussing your feelings with a trusted friend or family member? If so, who? If not, what would help you feel more comfortable?

----

2. What helps you calm down when you are upset?

----

3. How long do your emotions usually last? What causes them to change?

----

4. Have you ever avoided doing something because you were scared or nervous? If so, describe the situation.

----

5. Which emotions are the most difficult for you to manage?

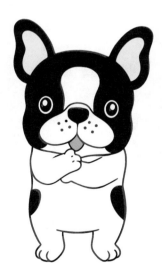

Activity 11
Labeling Your Emotions

When you go to the doctor because you're not feeling well, it helps if you can tell them exactly what's wrong. Simply saying, "I feel bad" will not help the doctor identify and treat the problem. It's similar with our emotions; we must recognize and label them before we can effectively manage them. Words like "stressed" or "upset" only communicate how you are feeling in a general way. It's more helpful if you can describe the stress or explain how you are feeling upset.

Psychologists have identified 5 basic emotions: anger, disgust, fear, happiness, and sadness. However, within these categories, there are multiple variations. For example, rage is a more extreme form of anger. Frustration is anger at not being able to accomplish something. Within the category of happiness, there are feelings like joy, excitement, and contentment.

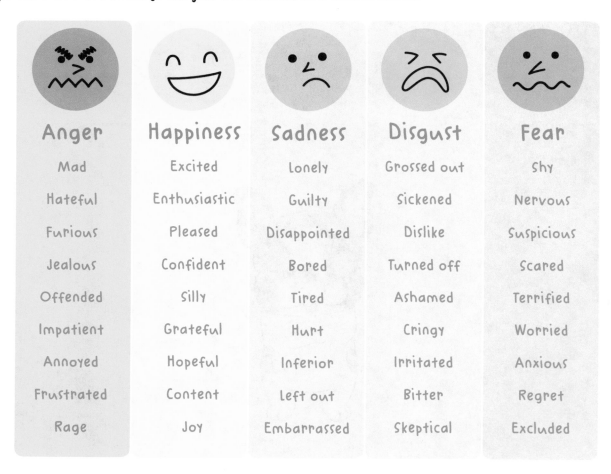

Anger	Happiness	Sadness	Disgust	Fear
Mad	Excited	Lonely	Grossed out	Shy
Hateful	Enthusiastic	Guilty	Sickened	Nervous
Furious	Pleased	Disappointed	Dislike	Suspicious
Jealous	Confident	Bored	Turned off	Scared
Offended	Silly	Tired	Ashamed	Terrified
Impatient	Grateful	Hurt	Cringy	Worried
Annoyed	Hopeful	Inferior	Irritated	Anxious
Frustrated	Content	Left out	Bitter	Regret
Rage	Joy	Embarrassed	Skeptical	Excluded

Use the feeling list to answer the following questions:

Can you think of something positive that happened recently? Describe the situation.

Which of the basic emotions did you experience?

Did you have any of the feeling variations listed under the basic emotions? If so, which ones?

What thoughts did you have when experiencing these emotions?

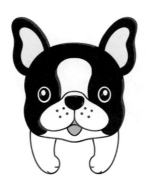

Now, do the same thing for a challenging situation:

What happened?

Which of the basic emotions did you experience?

Did you have any of the feeling variations listed under the basic emotions? If so, which ones?

What thoughts did you have when experiencing this emotion?

How did you feel about the feeling? (For example, justified in your anger versus ashamed of it)

What urges did you experience in connection with the emotion?

How did you behave as a result of the emotion?

Reflection:

How do you feel after completing this activity?

Did any of your answers surprise you? If so, which ones?

How can you use this information to better manage your emotions in future?

Activity 12
Checking the Facts

At this point, you may have noticed that thoughts, emotions, and behaviors are all connected. The way we think affects how we feel and behave, our emotions influence our behaviors, and so on. Thoughts, feelings, and behaviors are so interconnected, it can be difficult to figure out which came first! Did thinking about my long-lost friend make me feel sad, or did feeling sad cause me to think about my long-lost friend?

The good news is that changing your thoughts and/or behaviors can help regulate your emotions.

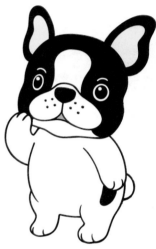

In this activity, we will practice checking the facts of a situation and revising our interpretations (thoughts) to change how we feel.

1. Think of a situation that is causing you to feel upset or uncomfortable. Which of the 5 basic emotions (anger, disgust, fear, happiness, sadness) is the cause?

----

2. How intense is this emotion from 1 (mild) to 10 (overwhelming)?

----

3. How long have you felt this way?

----

5. Were there other things going on, like being tired or hungry, that might have made the emotion worse?

----

6. Ask yourself. "Am I understanding the situation correctly?" What are the facts? What are your thoughts and opinions?

Example: I was worrying about being cut from the team before I even tried out.

----

7. What is the worst thing that could happen? How likely is it? How would you handle it if it actually happened?

Example: The worst thing that could happen is that I am cut and all my friends make it. This is not very likely because my friends and I are at the same skill level. If I get cut, I will be disappointed but I can use the extra time to practice and prepare for next season.

----

8. Do your feelings fit the facts of what happened? Is there another way to look at it?

Example: The feelings do not fit the facts. I have as much of a chance of making the team as any of my friends. I will be disappointed if I don't make it, but I will be okay.

----

9. After completing this activity, which of the following is most true? (Circle one)

   a) The emotion does not fit the facts of the situation, and I feel less angry/fearful/sad now.

   b) The emotion does not fit the facts, but I still feel angry/fearful/sad and need help to feel better.

   c) The emotion fits the facts, but the emotion is too intense and long-lasting and I need some more help.

   d) The emotion, intensity, and duration fit the facts, and I need a plan to handle it.

If you answered b, c, or d, you may be thinking, "But Ronny, I thought this activity was supposed to help me feel better. What now?" Sometimes, checking the facts of a situation is not enough to regulate our emotions. Similarly, there may be times when acting on your emotions is not the best course of action, even if they do fit the facts. If this is the case, you need to flip the script. Check out the next activity!

Activity 13
Flip the Script

Flipping the script means doing something in the opposite way that it is usually done. Just as changing your thoughts can affect how you feel, changing how you respond to a feeling can change the emotion itself.

When I am feeling sad, my instinct is to retreat to my doggie bed and hide from the world. But this usually does not help me to feel better. Alone in my bed, I have nothing to distract me from my thoughts, and I end up feeling sadder and lonelier. So, I challenge myself to flip the script and act in an opposite way to my emotions. Instead of wallowing in my sadness, I pick up a ball and go find my human for a game of fetch. My sadness might not disappear completely, but now it has to compete with other emotions like joy and love!

Let's brainstorm some opposite actions you could take when experiencing different emotions.

Anger

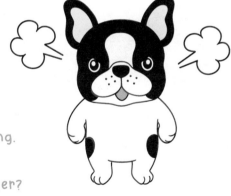

- Do something nice for the person you are angry with.
- Do a loving-kindness meditation (Activity 8) and direct it at the person who is making you angry.
- Use your energy for a fun activity like skating, biking, or swimming.

What ideas do you have for acting in an opposite way to your anger?

Fear

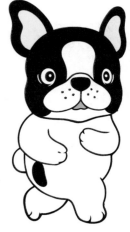

- Face your fear little by little.

    Imagine yourself approaching the scary place, activity, animal, or person. Use deep breathing to cope with any worries that come up. Then, confront the fear in real life, starting small and slowly spending more time with the scary thing as you feel more comfortable.

- Take actions that give you a sense of control in a scary situation.

    For example, if you're nervous about a party, see if you can help set up the snack table or play deejay.

- Look for signs that you are safe, like friendly faces or helpful adults.

- Pretend you're feeling brave! Stand tall with your head up and shoulders back and relaxed. Make eye contact and use a confident tone of voice.

What ideas do you have for acting in an opposite way to your fear?

Envy

- Count your blessings. Instead of focusing on what you don't have, list all the things you are grateful for.

- Check the facts to see if you are exaggerating either your difficulties or the blessings of the person you envy.

- Put yourself in the other person's shoes. What challenges might they be dealing with that you can't see?

- Stop the comparisons.

    Try not to compare yourself to others, especially on social media. Check your expectations to make sure they are realistic and not based on something that's impossible to achieve.

What ideas do you have for acting in an opposite way to envy?

Sadness

• Do the things you usually skip when you're feeling sad.

• Get active, whether this means exercise or completing a small task.

• Find the good in the present moment instead of getting carried away by negative thoughts.

What ideas do you have for acting in an opposite way to sadness?

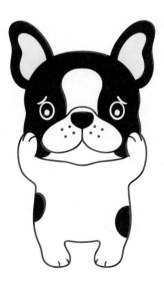

ABC Please

The next five activities relate to a group of DBT skills called "ABC PLEASE." Each letter stands for a skill that helps you manage your emotions and keeps you feeling your best. Here is a summary to help you remember the activities:

- Accumulate (build up) short- and long-term positive emotions
- Build mastery
- Cope ahead
- PLEASE skills
    - Treat Physical illness
    - Eat healthily
    - Avoid bad stuff
    - Get enough Sleep
    - Exercise

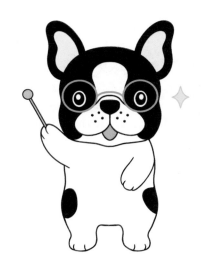

Activity 14

Accumulate Positive Emotions (Short-term)

Just as negative thoughts, emotions, and behaviors are all connected, the same goes for positive ones! When you are filled with positive emotions, you're more likely to have positive thoughts and behaviors, which then lead to more positive feelings. It's like a big loop of feeling good! And as if feeling good isn't motivation enough, research shows that positive emotions can help you fight off sickness and make tough times easier to handle.

One way you can accumulate (build up) positive emotions is by regularly doing fun activities. First, use the box below to brainstorm a list of interests, hobbies, and activities that bring you joy. These could be things you have done in the past or activities you have always wanted to try. Remember to include "small" things like listening to music, lying in the sun, or enjoying your favorite treat.

Now, choose one of these activities to do today.

Before starting the activity, rate your mood on a scale of 0 (terrible) to 10 (fantastic).

Use your mindfulness skills to fully engage in the activity. If your mind wanders to something else, gently refocus your attention on the present.

After completing the activity, again rate your mood. How did it change?

Repeat this process at least once a day, even if you are not in the mood. Prioritize it as you do other routine tasks like sleeping and brushing your teeth. Think of it as saving for a rainy day. The more positive emotions you accumulate (build up), the better able you will be to cope with life's challenges in the future!

Accumulate Positive Emotions (Long-term)

Fun activities help you accumulate (build up) positive emotions in the short term, but long-term happiness involves working towards goals, improving relationships, and having meaningful experiences. After all, a life well-lived is more than simply a collection of fun experiences.

Looking back on your life so far, what memories are most meaningful to you? Chances are, they involve overcoming a challenge, making a connection, or doing something that is really important to you. These experiences accumulate (build up) positive emotions like pride, gratitude, and self-worth.

To build these and other positive emotions, first identify a specific long-term goal.

This could be a school or sports achievement, to improve a relationship, or to make a difference in your community.

My goal: _____

Next, list the steps needed to achieve this goal. Make sure the steps are concrete and actionable. For example, instead of writing, "get good grades," think about how you would actually do this. "Study for an extra hour each day" or "Stay after school for extra help in math" are specific and attainable action steps.

Steps to achieve my goal:

1.——

2.——

3.——

4.——

5.——

Do something to work towards the first step. For example, you could set up a study area where you are unlikely to be distracted or interrupted.

Reflect on this experience:

Did you find yourself wanting to put it off? If so, why do you think that is? How did you overcome the urge to avoid? How did you feel after you took action?

——

——

——

Continue taking steps towards your goal, pausing to celebrate your achievements, however small. If self-criticism or self-doubt starts to creep in, "Check the Facts" (Activity 12) or "Flip the Script" (Activity 13)!

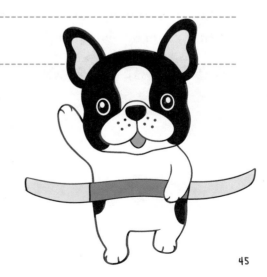

Activity 16
Building Mastery

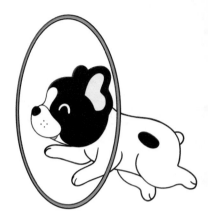

The most difficult trick I ever learned was jumping through a hoop. It was so hard to build up the courage to leap through that circle. It took some time for me to develop the coordination required, but once I mastered it, I felt like I could do anything! Even better, the memory of this accomplishment motivated me to try new tricks!

Mastering a challenging activity makes you feel happy and proud.

It also makes it easier to handle difficult situations in the future. Tricks not your thing? Fortunately, there are plenty of other ways you can build mastery.

Think about the times in your life when you've felt the most proud of yourself. What challenges did you face and how did you overcome them? Did you start with a smaller, more achievable task and work your way up to a bigger goal?

Using these past experiences, make a list of challenging but achievable tasks. If you need help, think about a skill you would like to develop. For example, if you want to improve your public speaking, your task could be giving a rehearsed speech to your family members.

Tasks I want to work on:

1. ....

2. ....

3. ....

Choose one task from your list and commit to achieving it. When, where, and how will you do it?

Task I choose: _____

When and where I will do it: _____

Steps I need to take:

1._____

2._____

3._____

4._____

5._____

If at first you don't succeed, try again with something just a little easier. If the task you chose is too easy for you, try something a little harder next time. Gradually increase the difficulty of the task until you feel you've mastered it. Then, move on to another challenging task!

Bonus Activity

After you complete a task, take a moment to reflect by answering the following questions.

How did it feel to complete the task?

_____

_____

What emotions did you experience? List both positive and negative.

How did this task help you build confidence?

Activity 17

Cope Ahead of Time with Difficult Situations

I love to go on walks with my human, but this was not always the case. You see, there's a big German Shepherd dog that lives on our street, and every time my human and I walk by, he barks like he wants to eat me for breakfast! My human told me that he was just protecting his house, but I still got super scared every time we got near him. It got so bad I didn't even want to go on walks anymore!

Eventually, I decided not to let my fear prevent me from doing something that I love. I came up with a list of things that I could do to cope with the situation.

For example, I could guide my human to the other side of the street to create some distance between me and the Shepherd.

Coping ahead of time with the scary German Shepherd was way more effective than avoiding the situation entirely. Avoiding not only stops you from doing things you want to do but can also make the emotion more powerful in the end.

To practice coping ahead, first think of a situation that might upset you or make you behave in a way that you don't want.

Imagine the situation in as much detail as possible. Really immerse yourself in it and try to feel the emotions you would feel if it were happening in real life.

What is the situation?

Who is involved, and where does it take place?

What emotions might be triggered that make it difficult to cope?

How might you behave in the situation without an action plan?

Now, decide which coping or problem-solving skills you want to use. If you need help, refer to Activity 13, "Flip the Script." How might you act differently in order to achieve a different result? For me, this meant approaching the German Shepherd instead of avoiding him.

My chosen coping skills:

What will you do to manage any negative emotions that come up? I decided I would take lots of deep breaths to signal to my body that there was nothing to fear.

My plan for managing negative emotions:

Now, imagine yourself using your chosen coping skills to manage the situation effectively. What effect might that have?

Finally, take some deep breaths or use another relaxation technique to calm your body down. Practice this until you feel you can confront the situation in real life.

Activity 18

PLEASE—Taking Care of Your Mind by Taking Care of Your Body

I'm a pretty happy pup, but every once in a while, I get cranky. I've noticed this tends to happen more when I am tired, hungry, or not feeling well. When my body's not feeling well, it's hard for my mind to feel well.

Your mind and body are connected and in constant communication. What affects one, affects the other. So if your goal is to manage your emotions more effectively, you've got to take care of your body first.

In this activity, we will practice caring for your physical health to improve your emotional health. The letters in the word "PLEASE" stand for activities that help you feel better physically and mentally.

Treat Physical illness — If you're sick, take any medicines your doctor has given you and take it easy until you feel better.

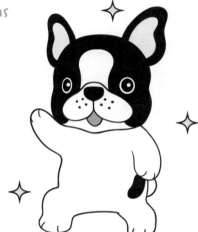

Eat healthily — Give your body a variety of foods to keep it strong and healthy. Candy, sweets, and things with artificial colors and flavors may taste good, but too much can make you feel yucky in both your body and mind.

Avoid bad stuff — Stay away from junk food, drugs, alcohol, caffeine, and sugar, as these things can mess with your mood.

Get enough Sleep — Aim for at least 8 hours of sleep per night. Having a bedtime routine and shutting off screens after a certain time can help with this.

Exercise — Play outside, ride your bike, participate in a sport, or do something active every day.

What is one thing you want to do to start taking better care of your body?

Examples include eating a fruit or vegetable at every meal, going for a walk (take your dog if you have one!), or cutting back on sugar.

Part 3
Distress Tolerance

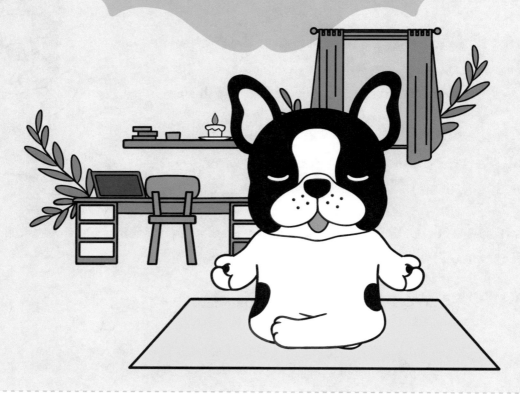

Congratulations on finishing Part 2 of this workbook! The emotion regulation skills will help you manage your emotions and keep you feeling good in your mind and body. Of course, even if you become a master emotion regulator, you will still experience negative emotions on occasion. Anxiety, stress, sadness, frustration, and anger are part of life.

That's where distress tolerance comes in.

Distress tolerance is the ability to sit with uncomfortable feelings instead of acting on them and making things worse.

The skills in this section are not permanent solutions to your problems, but short-term coping skills to help you through difficult situations. It's a little like treating the symptom versus the root cause.

Let me explain with a personal experience:

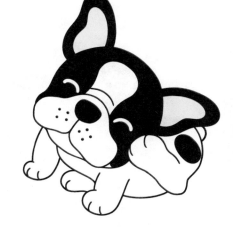

Like most dogs, I use my back legs to scratch myself when I have an itch. Usually, it's underneath my collar or behind my ears. But a few years ago, I was itchy all over! No matter how long and hard I scratched, the itch just wouldn't go away. My human tried giving me oatmeal baths, which helped for a while, but the itch always came back. Finally, we went to the vet. It turned out to be fleas! The vet gave us a special shampoo to use, and the itching went away for good.

The oatmeal baths treated the symptom, but the anti-flea shampoo treated the cause of the itching. Likewise, distress tolerance skills treat the symptoms but not the cause of the distress. So make sure you eventually deal with the source of the negative emotions; otherwise, they are likely to return!

Use distress tolerance skills when:

- You're feeling really upset and don't know how to fix it.
- Your emotions are giving you the urge to do something that is likely to make things worse.
- You are in emotion mind and need to calm down before you can think clearly.

Activity 19
Stress Survey

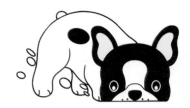

The purpose of this survey is to explore when, where, and how you experience distress. By under-standing the circumstances around your distress, you can cope ahead with the right skills.

1. How often do you experience distress in a normal week?

----

2. What are the main causes of this distress?

----

3. List three strategies you've used to cope with this distress.

    a. _____ Was it helpful? (Yes, No, Somewhat)

    b. _____ Was it helpful? (Yes, No, Somewhat)

    c. _____ Was it helpful? (Yes, No, Somewhat)

4. Does your distress interfere with your life? If so, how?

----

5. Are there times of the year when you are more likely to experience distress?

Activity 20

STOP!

Have you ever played freeze tag? It's like regular tag except that when you get tagged you have to freeze in your current position until someone unfreezes you. This distress tolerance activity is a little like playing freeze tag with your emotions.

The idea is to "freeze" long enough to decide what to do, instead of acting impulsively on your emotions.

You can remember the steps of this activity with the acronym "STOP."

Stop —Freeze! Do not move a muscle. Imagine your emotions are attracted to movement, and as long as you stay perfectly still, they cannot take control!

Take a step back — Take a break. If possible, physically remove yourself from the situation. Take a few deep breaths.

Observe — Notice what is going on around you as well as inside of you. Describe the facts of the situation. How are the facts different from your thoughts and feelings?

Proceed mindfully — Ask your wise mind how you should proceed. Which actions will make the situation better or worse?

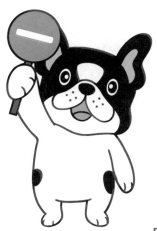

The next time you feel overwhelmed by negative emotions, STOP the cycle of negative thoughts, feelings, and behaviors! Then, use the questions on the next page to record your observations.

1. What was the situation?

----

2. What emotions were involved?

----

3. What urges did you experience?

----

4. Were you able to take a break from the situation? How?

----

5. What observations did you make after taking a step back?

6.How did you proceed? Did you use mindfulness or any other skills?

----

7. How did you feel afterward?

Activity 21
All Aboard the Decision Train!
Using Pros and Cons to Decide Between Two Courses of Action

Strong emotional urges are like a runaway train, rumbling down the track at top speed. You are the conductor and you have to decide whether to put the brakes on or let the train go and risk disaster.

Putting on the brakes involves resisting the urge, which may be uncomfortable in the short term but lets you act mindfully and effectively in the long term. Letting the train continue down the track may feel good in the short term but often carries with it unwanted consequences.

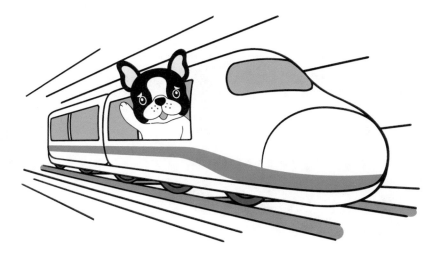

Think of a situation in which you had the urge to act impulsively and answer the following questions:

What was the situation?

_____

_____

What emotions were involved? _____

What was the urge? _____

Now, list the pros and cons of acting on the urge and the pros and cons of resisting the urge.

Here is an example:

Situation: Humans baking delicious cookies in the oven

Emotion: Desire

Urge: Sneak a cookie while they are cooling on the rack

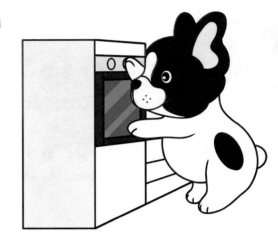

	Pros	Importance Rating	Cons	Importance Rating
Acting on the urge	The cookie would be delicious	2	The humans would be mad	4
	My craving would be satisfied	3	I might burn my mouth	5
			I might be punished	4
			I would feel guilty afterward	5
Resisting the urge	The humans would be happy	5	My mouth would continue to water	2
	I would not be risking hurting myself	5	I might need to use some skills to cope with my discomfort	4
	I would feel good about myself	5		

Notice how I have also rated each pro and con on a scale from 1 (very little importance) to 5 (high importance). This information will help you make the best, wise-mind choice. One thing I realized when I did this activity is that the pros of acting on my urge are short-term while the cons are longer-lasting. And the pros of resisting the urge include important things like sticking to my values, while the cons are just discomfort for a short amount of time.

Now it's your turn! Try filling out the grid below when you are in a wise-mind state. Over time, you will learn to put up with uncomfortable urges and other types of distress without engaging in behaviors that hurt you in the long run!

Situation: _____

Emotion: _____

Urge: _____

	Pros	Importance Rating	Cons	Importance Rating
Acting on the urge				
Resisting the urge				

Activity 22

TIPP-ing the Scales of Distress

I don't know about you, but when I am in distress (upset), it's hard to think straight and make good, wise-mind choices. Even when I try to STOP and carry on mindfully, my emotions continue to derail me! When this happens, I "TIPP" the scales of my distress, calming my body to reduce the intensity of negative emotions.

If you've ever watched a science experiment, you know that chemical reactions can happen very quickly. TIPP can work quickly, too. That's because it changes your body chemistry to help you feel calmer.

Before we get started, it's important to see your doctor if you have any medical issues or are taking medications that may affect how you respond to this activity.

Like many of the other skills in this workbook, TIPP is an acronym, with each letter representing a different activity.

Temperature

- To use this skill, prepare a bowl of cold water or a zip-lock bag filled with cold water.
- Take a deep breath and hold it.
- Put your face in the cold water or place the bag on your eyes and cheeks.
- Hold for 15–30 seconds then slowly remove your face from the water and breathe out.
- Notice the effects on your body and emotions.
- Do this again if you need to calm down more.

Intense exercise

- Choose a physical activity, such as running, doing jumping jacks, or dancing.

- Do this activity intensely (using lots of energy) for several minutes.

- Notice the effects on your body and emotions.

- If you are still feeling upset, do the activity for a bit longer.

Paced breathing

- Slow the pace of your breathing by breathing in for 5 seconds and breathing out for 7 seconds. Do this for several minutes.

- Notice the effects on your body and emotions.

- Repeat this activity until you feel more relaxed.

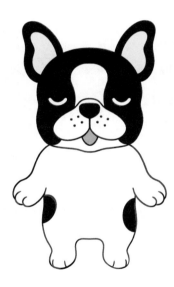

Paired muscle relaxation

- Get into a comfortable position, either sitting or lying down.

- Starting with your face, tense and relax the following muscles. Hold the tension for several seconds while you breathe in, then relax as you breathe out.

- Tense the muscles in your forehead, mouth, and jaw. Scrunch up your lips towards your nose and your nose towards your eyes. Clench your jaw. Release.

- Tense the muscles in your neck and shoulders. Raise your shoulders towards your ears. Hold for several seconds, then release.

- Tense the muscles in your back by arching your back and bringing your shoulder blades together. Release.

- Tense your chest by taking a deep breath and holding it. Let go if it becomes uncomfortable or difficult.

- Tense your arms and hands by making tight fists and bending both arms up to touch your shoulders. Squeeze, then release.

- Tense your stomach by tightening your tummy muscles as if you are preparing for a punch. Hold for several seconds, then release.

- Tense your legs by stretching them out in front of you, squeezing your thighs together, and bending your feet. Release.

- Tense your ankles and feet by stretching your legs out in front of you, curling your toes, and bending your feet. Release.

- Feel if you have any remaining tension in your body and repeat the exercise if you need to.

- Rest for 1 minute, breathing deeply and enjoying the feeling of relaxation.

Note that you don't need to do all of the TIPP activities at once; choose an activity to start with, and then add another activity if you still feel upset!

Activity 23
Distracting with ACCEPTS

We generally think of distractions as a bad thing, but sometimes it can be helpful to distract yourself, like when you are feeling overwhelmed with negative emotions. There are many ways to do this. Personally, I prefer to go for a walk with my human or roll around in the grass. Remember to use your mindfulness skills to fully engage in the activity!

You can remember this skill with the acronym ACCEPTS. Here are some ideas you can try:

Activities: Enjoy a non-stressful activity. Read a book, call a friend, watch a movie, play a game, listen to music, draw, or paint.

Contributions: Do something nice for someone else. Complete a chore without being asked, do a favor, help a friend with homework, volunteer, or donate money or other items.

Comparisons: Compare yourself to those who might have it harder than you. Note that this doesn't mean you "shouldn't" feel the way you do, just that you have blessings as well as challenges.

Emotions: Do something that makes you feel a different emotion than the one you're feeling now. Watch a funny movie if you are feeling sad, listen to calming music if you are feeling anxious, or write a thank-you note if you are feeling angry.

Push away: For a short amount of time, push your problems out of your mind. Imagine putting your worries in a box on a high shelf in a closet or build an imaginary wall between you and the problem.

Thoughts: Fill your head with other thoughts. Sing your favorite song, read a funny comic strip, play Sudoku or do a crossword puzzle.

Sensations: Distract yourself with physical sensations. Blast music, take a hot or cold shower, squeeze a stress ball, hold an ice cube in your hand, or cuddle up in a soft blanket.

Choose one of the above activities to use the next time you are in a upsetting situation.

Which activity will you try?

After completing the activity, answer the following questions:

Did the activity help you put up with being upset and/or your urges?

Were you able to avoid acting without thinking first and making the situation worse? If yes, congratulations! If not, go easy on yourself and try again with another ACCEPTS activity. Sometimes, you need lots of skills to put up with a painful situation, and not every skill is going to work for you every time.

Activity 24
Self-soothing with 5 Senses

Remember in Part I of this workbook when we used our 5 senses to become more mindful of everyday experiences? In this activity, we are going to use our senses to help us put up with being upset so that we can feel better.

Think of it as a "mini vacation" from your problems!

One of my favorite memories is going on a hike with my human. There were so many new things to see, hear, smell, taste, and touch! I especially loved the sound of the stream that ran alongside the trail and the taste of the cool water on my tongue. Now, whenever I feel overwhelmed, I put on some soothing nature sounds and take a refreshing drink of water.

Here are some other ideas for self-soothing with your 5 senses:

Soothing SIGHTS
- Pretty pictures or other artwork
- Photographs that remind you of happy memories
- The colors outside your window
- A fun toy like a kaleidoscope or snow globe

Soothing SOUNDS
- Your favorite music
- A calming meditation
- The sound of your favorite musical instrument

Soothing SMELLS
- Your favorite lotion, body wash, or shampoo
- A nice-smelling candle
- Essential oils like lavender, vanilla, etc.
- Flowers

Soothing TASTES
- A yummy cup of tea or hot cocoa
- Freshly baked cookies

Soothing things to TOUCH
- A soft, furry blanket
- A bubble bath
- A worry stone or fidget toy

What are some ways you can use your 5 senses to feel better?

Activity 25

Improving the Moment

How was your mini vacation? Did you feel better after using your 5 senses? Sometimes, even after using your senses or the ACCEPTS skills, you need a little extra help putting up with being upset. That's where IMPROVE comes in!

IMPROVE skills are another toolkit you can use during tough times. They are particularly helpful when it seems like there's no way out or the challenges just won't stop.

As with many of the other activities in this workbook, each letter of the word IMPROVE stands for a specific skill.

Imagery — Imagine a relaxing scene. Create a fantasy world in your mind, one where your problems magically disappear. Think back to a happier time and imagine you are reliving it.

Meaning — See if you can find some meaning in your current experience. For example, maybe your current challenges will make you stronger and tougher in the future.

Prayer — Ask God, a higher power, or your own wise mind for the strength to handle being upset, trusting that they have a plan for you and will help guide you through difficult moments.

Relaxation — Breathe deeply and relax your muscles. Do some light stretching or self-massage. Fix your mouth in a half-smile. Hum a relaxing tune.

One thing in the moment — Focus all of your attention on what you are doing in the moment. Watch out for and accept any physical sensations without judgment. Notice when your mind wanders and gently bring it back to the present.

Vacation — Give yourself a break. Go outside, take a walk, or splash some cold water on your face. Plan a day off from school or a fun weekend with friends. Unplug or power down your devices. Do a short meditation.

Encouragement — Talk to yourself as you would a close friend. Be your own cheerleader with statements like "You've got this!" Remind yourself that you are doing the best that you can in the situation and that it won't last forever.

Which skill did you find the most helpful?

Which did you find the most challenging?

How can you use IMPROVE in your everyday life?

Activity 26
Radical Acceptance

There's an old saying that goes, "Pain is inevitable, but suffering is optional." In other words, pain is a part of life but we don't have to suffer because of it. Now, you might be thinking, Ronny, it's not like I want to suffer. If I could avoid it, I would. Well, I'm going to teach you how to do just that with a skill called radical acceptance.

You see, suffering has two parts—pain and resistance. The pain is uncomfortable, but the resistance to the pain is what causes long-term suffering. Let me explain with a story:

A few years ago, our yard was overrun with dandelions. My human and I would spend hours pulling them up by the roots only to have them sprout somewhere else. We spread special fertilizer and treated the lawn with weed control, but nothing helped. Finally, we called a lawn care expert, who said he could help us with our problem. We were so excited, we told him we would do whatever he advised! He said, "I advise that you learn to accept those dandelions."

The dandelions weren't the problem. Our resistance to the dandelions was the problem. Once we learned to radically accept the dandelions, our suffering ceased. We learned to appreciate the lawn for what it was—mostly lush and green, but with some weeds mixed in.

Radical acceptance is accepting the facts of a situation even if they are disappointing.

Radical acceptance doesn't mean you have to agree with what is happening, or that you need to "give up" trying to improve the situation. With radical acceptance, you accept reality in the short term so that you can do what is necessary later on. It's willingness versus willfulness.

Willingness is:

- Enjoying life even though it's sometimes painful
- Making the most of life even if you can't have everything you want in every situation
- Doing what works instead of focusing on what you wish were happening

Willfulness is:

- Refusing to accept the facts of a situation
- Trying to control every part of your life
- Giving up because you can't have exactly what you want

Here are some examples of willfulness and willingness:

Situation	Willful	Willing
You are at sports practice and you feel a sharp pain in your ankle.	You keep practicing because you want to play in the next game.	You tell your coach about the pain so you can avoid further injury.
You are excited to see the new Disney movie but your friends want to see the Marvel movie.	You stay home because you can't see the movie you want to see.	You go along with your friends because it is still fun to hang out, even if it's not your first choice of movie.
You are invited to a friend's birthday party but it's at the same time as a family celebration.	You refuse to talk to anyone at the family celebration, instead checking your phone for updates on your friend's party.	You are disappointed to miss your friend's party but try to distract yourself by catching up with family members you haven't seen in a while.

Describe a situation when you acted willfully:

How did it turn out?

Here is a step-by-step guide to practicing willingness and radical acceptance:

1. Notice when you are acting willful. (Hint: willful actions often come with thoughts like, "It's not fair!" or "It shouldn't be this way!")

2. Remember that you can't change the facts of the situation. Tell yourself, "This is how it is right now."

3. Commit to accepting the situation.

4. Practice this acceptance with your whole self, using the techniques in Activity 27, "Flip the script" (Activity 13), or "Cope Ahead" (Activity 17).

5. Watch out for any physical sensations or negative emotions.

6. Remind yourself that life is enjoyable even when there is pain or disappointment.

7. Make a list of the pros and cons of approaching the situation with willingness versus willfulness.

Activity 27
Techniques for Practicing Radical Acceptance

What did you think of the radical acceptance activity? What thoughts, feelings, and behaviors come with accepting reality? What thoughts, feelings, and behaviors come with resisting it?

Radical acceptance is hard. In fact, it might be the hardest skill in this workbook! Luckily, there are some tricks that can help you accept reality with your whole self—body and mind.

To practice radical acceptance with the body, try the following:

HALF-SMILE: Relax the muscles in your face, then slightly lift the corners of your mouth in a barely noticeable smile. Use a calm, peaceful expression. Remember, your body (including your face) communicates to your mind!

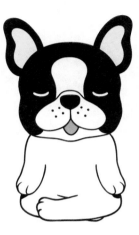

WILLING HANDS: Sit quietly and place your hands on your lap, palms facing up. Relax your muscles from shoulders to fingertips. Imagine yourself accepting reality and letting go of resistance.

You can also put these two skills together to practice radical acceptance of a challenging person:

- Think of a person who makes you feel angry or upset.
- Take a few deep breaths, then fix your mouth in a half-smile.
- Relax your hands and turn your palms up.
- Picture the person that is causing you to suffer.
- Think about this person's experience.
    - What makes them happy or sad?
    - What do they think and feel?
    - What are their hopes and values?
    - Are they influenced by things like prejudice or anger?
    - What past experiences may be affecting their behavior?
    - Are they fully in control of their actions?
- Continue until you feel your negative emotion being replaced by compassion.
- Repeat this several times for the same person before moving on to someone new.

To practice radical acceptance with the mind, TURN YOUR MIND:

- Imagine you are walking down an empty street. You come to a fork in the road. One "branch" is the rejection road and one is the acceptance road.
- Along the rejection road are willfulness, resistance, and suffering.
- Along the acceptance road are willingness, mindful action, and peace.
- Imagine choosing to walk down the acceptance road.
- Picture yourself walking the path to acceptance and leaving resistance behind.

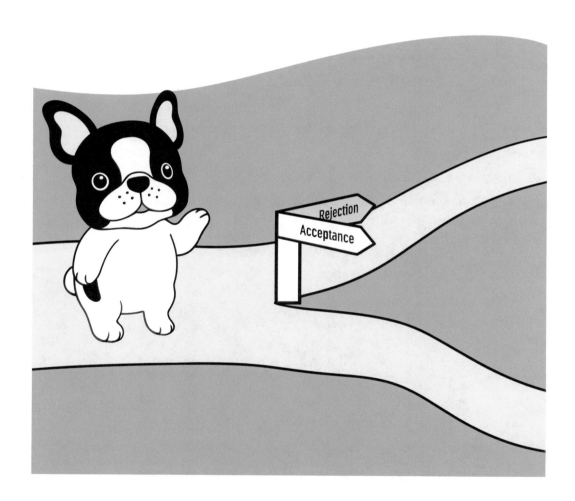

Part 4
Interpersonal Effectiveness

Welcome to the last part of this workbook! ! Take a moment to think about how far you have come. Which activities have you found to be the most helpful? Which skills are still a bit tricky for you?

This final section is all about relationships—building them, keeping them going, and dealing with conflict. Connecting with others is one of life's most rewarding experiences, but it's not always easy. Miscommunications, misunderstandings, and emotion mind can all get in the way.

For example, a few summers ago, we had a heat wave. I wear a fur coat 24/7, so I was sweltering! My human doesn't like me going swimming because then I need a bath, and you know how I feel about baths. One day, we went for a walk along a river. The water looked so refreshing, I jumped right in! I put my immediate urge (cooling off) ahead of my long-term goal of respecting my human's wishes. If only I could have told my human how I was feeling and avoided resorting to impulsive behavior!

The skills in this section will help you get what you want when talking to people, whether that's understanding, permission to do something, being taken seriously, or avoiding conflict. But more importantly, these skills will help you improve your relationships and keep your self-respect!

Activity 28
Relationship Reflection

How do you feel when you are around other people? Are there certain situations that are difficult to manage? Understanding how you feel and act in your relationships is the first step towards getting better at them! The questions in this activity will help you understand your relationship strengths, goals, and areas for improvement.

"Circle the answer that sounds most like you!"

1. How do you generally feel when communicating with family and friends?

   · Comfortable / Anxious

   · Confident / Insecure

   · Respected / Disrespected

   · Other: _____

2. How often do you have disagreements or arguments with family and friends?

   All the time   Sometimes   Rarely   Never

3. How easy or difficult is it for you to express your needs to other people, such as asking for help or saying no to something you don't want to do?

   Very Easy   Easy   Difficult   Very Difficult

4. How easy or difficult is it for you to listen carefully when others are speaking?

   Very Easy   Easy   Difficult   Very Difficult

   If it's difficult, why?: _____

5. How often do you speak up and express how you feel when someone upsets you?

All the time	Sometimes	Rarely	Never

6. How often do you make assumptions about other people—for example, assuming that they don't like you?

All the time	Sometimes	Rarely	Never

7. Think about one time when you felt proud of how you spoke to someone in a difficult situation.

I felt proud when:

_____

_____

8. Which friends or family members do you most admire for how they communicate with others?

I admire: _____ because_____

_____

9. What are your goals for this part of the workbook?

My goals are:

_____

_____

Express Yourself!
Exploring Communication Styles

Communication is all about sharing our thoughts, feelings, and ideas. Sometimes we do it with words, sometimes with actions, and sometimes with body language and facial expressions. While there is no wrong way to express yourself, certain communication styles tend to be better than others for making sure everyone feels heard and respected. Let's check out the different styles:

- Passive communication—Rather than saying what you feel or think, you try to hide your emotions because you are scared of upsetting others. You may also feel like your opinions don't matter as much as other people's. This makes it hard for you to get your needs met because you don't speak up.

- Aggressive communication—You express your feelings directly, but in not-so-nice ways. You might try to control other people in order to get what you want even if it harms them in some way. This causes people to not want to be around you sometimes.

- Passive-aggressive communication—You don't say what you feel directly, but instead express yourself with sarcasm or other negative behaviors. You might say one thing when you mean another, give someone the silent treatment, or purposely "forget" to fulfill your promises.

- Assertive communication—You are honest but respectful. You say what you think and feel in a clear, direct manner, but also listen to other people so you can understand their points of view. You work together to find solutions that make everyone feel valued and respected.

Which communication style do you use the most often?

It's okay to have a mix of styles, but assertive communication tends to work best. Being more assertive in your relationships can help you get along better with others and feel better about yourself at the same time!

Decide whether the following communications are passive, aggressive, passive-aggressive, or assertive:

I thought you were a snob at first, but you're actually cool.	I understand your point of view. Can I explain my perspective?	Oh great, I get to sit next to you! (When you don't like the person)
It's nothing. (When something is bothering you)	I'll tell everyone your secret unless you do this for me.	I can't help with the project tonight. Can we do it tomorrow?
When you blow off our plans, I feel frustrated and unimportant.	I'll do whatever you want to do. (When you have a preference)	You aren't going to come with us? You're such a baby!

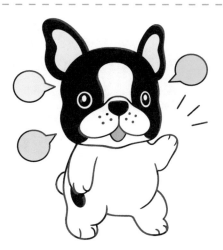

Activity 30

Be more Assertive with DEAR MAN

Want to communicate more assertively, but don't know how? This activity will help you express your needs and wants in a respectful, assertive way. When used properly, DEAR MAN can make it more likely for you to get what you want out of talking to someone. It can be used to ask for something, to say no when someone asks you for something, or to resolve an argument.

Have you ever needed something from someone but felt too scared to ask? Have you ever felt uncomfortable saying no to something you didn't want to do? Have you ever been "talked into" changing your point of view because you didn't know how to express yourself properly? DEAR MAN can help you in all of these situations, without having to use aggressive (yelling or blaming) or passive (unclear or non-direct) communication styles!

Can you think of a future situation when you will need to ask for something, say no to someone, or settle an argument?

Using DEAR MAN and the chart below, write down what you want to say. After you've completed the chart, practice in front of a mirror as if you were talking to the person in real life.

Describe: Say what happened. Just the facts! For example: You didn't come home when you said you would.	

Express: Share your feelings and opinions. Don't assume the other person knows how you feel or how the situation makes you feel.

For example: When you break a promise, I feel like you don't care about me.

_____

_____

_____

_____

_____

_____

Assert: Ask for what you want. Be clear and specific. Remember that other people cannot read your mind.

For example: I would like you to respect my feelings by doing what you say you're going to do.

_____

_____

_____

_____

_____

_____

Reinforce ahead of time: Explain what's in it for the other person if they do what you ask. You can also note any negative consequences of not meeting your needs.

For example: If you do this, I will feel happier and more relaxed around you, and we can have more fun together. If you continue to break your promises, I won't want to make plans with you.

_____

_____

_____

_____

Stay Mindful: Stay focused on your goal. Try not to get distracted or let the other person change the subject. Be a "broken record," repeating your request calmly, if necessary.

For example: We are not talking about times in the past when I have disappointed you. We are talking about your broken promise. I need to be able to trust that you will do what you say.

_____
_____
_____
_____
_____
_____

Appear Confident: Even if you don't feel confident, look like you are! Make eye contact, stand up straight, and speak clearly. Avoid apologies or uncertain statements.

For example: I value your feelings and I hope that you value mine.

_____
_____
_____
_____
_____

Negotiate: If the person says no, be willing to compromise. Offer alternative solutions or ask for their input.

For example: Would it help if I reminded you of our plans the day before?

_____
_____
_____
_____

Activity 31

GIVE to Get

Getting what you want out of talking to someone is wonderful, but not if it leaves your friend feeling hurt or angry. This next set of skills will help you balance your personal goals with the long-term health of the relationship. You can remember the skills with the acronym GIVE:

Be Gentle: Talk to your friends with kindness and respect. Use a gentle tone of voice. Avoid yelling or saying mean things. Instead, use "I" statements to explain how you feel. I statements focus on your thoughts and opinions instead of your friends' behavior.

Try it: Think of a time when you felt upset with a friend. Write down how you could talk to them in a gentle way. Use "I" statements like "I feel..." or "I need...".

Example: "I felt hurt when you borrowed my toy without asking. I need you to ask me first next time."

Now it's your turn: _____

_____

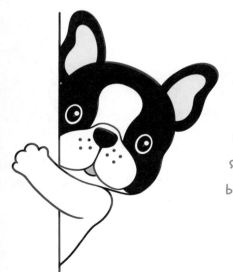

Act Interested: Give the other person your undivided attention. Listen to what they have to say without interrupting. Show that you care about what they are saying by leaning forward, making eye contact, and uncrossing your arms and legs. Be patient and sensitive to the other person's needs—for example, if they need a break from the conversation.

Validate: Show the other person that you understand and accept their thoughts, feelings, and actions, even if you don't agree with them. Try to see things from their point of view.

Try it: Think of a time when your friend shared their feelings with you, then answer the following questions:

What did they say?_____

_____

What is one possible answer that shows you understand how they feel?

Example: "I understand that you felt left out when we played without you. It makes sense that you're upset."

_____

_____

If you are feeling stuck, try beginning your answer with one of these validating phrases:

- If I'm hearing you correctly...

- It's understandable that...

- It sounds like...

Use an Easy Manner: Make the conversation comfortable by smiling and staying relaxed. Tell a joke if it feels right and keep your body language calm.

The next time you need to ask for something, say no when a friend asks you something, or sort out an argument, think about how you would like your friendship to be in the future. How do you want your friend to feel after talking with you? What skills do you need to use to keep and improve the friendship?

Activity 32
The FAST Track to Self-respect

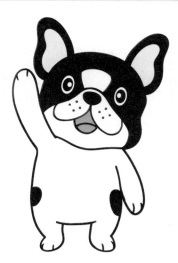

So far, we've learned how to get your needs met in a way that makes the other person feel respected and valued. But what about self-respect? Self-respect means feeling proud of how you handled a situation. Without self-respect, you risk feeling disappointed, ashamed, embarrassed, or worried. Let me give you an example:

One time, I was working on a group project at school. I was really excited because the project was about dinosaurs, and I love dinosaurs! I had so many great ideas, but my classmates just kept ignoring me. I was so frustrated, I felt like screaming! But instead, I used my FAST skills to speak up in a way that got their attention but also made me feel good about how I handled the situation.

Here is an overview of the FAST skills:

Be Fair: Don't sacrifice your feelings and needs to please others. Remember that your ideas and experiences are just as valid as the other person's.

Don't Over-Apologize: Don't apologize for speaking up. Remember it's okay to have different opinions than other people. Act confident and try not to slump or look at the floor.

Stick to Values: Stay true to what you think is right, even in challenging situations.

Be Truthful: Be honest. Avoid lying, acting helpless, exaggerating, or making excuses.

I knew that my ideas would help the group with the dinosaur project. So, I used my FAST skills:

Be Fair: I made sure my ideas were heard by politely getting my classmates' attention, showing that my thoughts were just as important as theirs.

Don't Over-Apologize: I spoke up confidently without saying "sorry" for having ideas, because it's okay to have different opinions.

Stick to Values: I stuck to my value that everyone deserves to be heard, and I made sure my voice was included in the project.

Be Truthful: I honestly explained my ideas and shared how I felt frustrated about being ignored at first.

Now it's your turn! Think of a time when might have to stand up for yourself or share your ideas. How will you use the FAST skills?

Be Fair: How will you make sure your feelings and needs are respected?

Don't Over-Apologize: What will you say to express yourself clearly and respectfully without apologizing too much?

Stick to Values: What values will you stick to? (For example, equality, respect)

Be Truthful: How will you be honest about how you feel and why your needs are important?

Remember, FAST skills help you feel good about how you've spoken to people. With FAST, you can talk to people more confidently and leave them feeling satisfied!

Activity 33
Think Skill

What do you think about the skills we've learned so far in this section? Which one has helped you the most? Are there any skills you continue to find tricky?

When someone has hurt or angered you in some way, it can be hard to stop and think about the best way to handle the situation. Your immediate urge might be to lash out or defend yourself in some way. While this is normal, it often makes the problem worse in the end.

In this activity, we are going to learn how to handle disagreements with kindness and curiosity instead of anger and defensiveness. We can do this with a group of skills called THINK:

Stop and Think: Take a deep breath. If possible, take a break from the disagreement until you can approach it mindfully.

Have Empathy: Imagine how the other person may be feeling.

Interpretations: List three to five possible explanations for the other person's behavior. Include at least one explanation in which the other person meant no harm.

Notice: Think of times when the other person was kind to you.

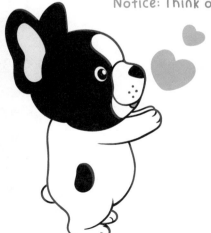

Use Kindness: Using all the relationship skills that you've learned so far, write a script of what you can say to the other person that would show kindness, empathy, and an open mind.

Use the chart below to explore how you can use THINK to manage disagreements with kindness and curiosity!

Steps	Your own experience	Example
Stop and Think	Write about a time when you disagreed with someone and things got heated. What happened? _____ _____ _____ _____ How did you react? _____ _____ _____ What do you think would have happened if you were able to stop and take a breath before reacting? _____ _____ _____ _____	I was playing a game with a friend and we disagreed about the rules. Suddenly, my friend shouted at me and called me a cheater. Instead of shouting back, I took a deep breath and thought about why they might be upset.

Steps	Your own experience	Example
Have Empathy	How might the other person have been feeling? ------------------------------ ------------------------------ ------------------------------ ------------------------------ ------------------------------	My friend could have been feeling frustrated or confused about the rules. If they really thought I was cheating, they could have been feeling hurt and disrespected.
Interpretations	Can you think of three to five possible explanations for the other person's behavior? Include at least one explanation in which the other person meant no harm. ------------------------------ ------------------------------ ------------------------------ ------------------------------ ------------------------------ ------------------------------	1. My friend was having a bad day. 2. My friend was hungry or tired and that made it harder for them to manage their emotions. 3. My friend was angry about something that didn't have anything to do with the game.

Steps	Your own experience	Example
Notice	Write about a time when the other person did something kind for you. ------------------------------ ------------------------------ ------------------------------ ------------------------------ ------------------------------ ------------------------------	My friend and I were playing a different game, and they let me have a "do over" when I didn't like what happened on my first try.
Use Kindness	Write down a kind and understanding response you could use next time. ------------------------------ ------------------------------ ------------------------------ ------------------------------ ------------------------------	I understand you might be frustrated, but when you call me names, it hurts my feelings. Do you want to take a snack break and come back to the game later?

Activity 34
Interpersonal Mindfulness

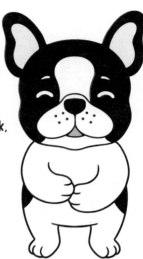

Hopefully you remember your mindfulness skills from Part I of this workbook, but if not—don't worry! Here is a little reminder:

Mindfulness means:
- paying attention to what you're doing right now
- accepting your thoughts, feelings, and urges without judgment

We can use mindfulness to pay attention and be present when talking to others. This helps us communicate and get along better. Mindfulness can also turn down the volume on emotion mind so you can make wise-mind decisions about how to handle situations with friends and family.

Now, let's practice being mindful when talking to someone. Read through the tips below. Then, talk with a family member, friend, or teacher and use these tips to stay mindful. Afterward, write what happened in the spaces below.

1. Pay attention—Focus on the person you're talking to. Notice their words, actions, and expressions. What are two things you noticed?

----

2. Focus on the present— Don't think about what you are going to say next. How did you help yourself stay focused? (For example, using the 5 senses, putting away distractions like toys or electronics)

----

3. Let go of judgments—If you start thinking something like "This is boring" or "I don't like this," let that thought drift away like a boat on a stream.

Write down one judgmental thought you had and how you let it go:

• Thought: _____

• How I let it go: _____

4. Join in fully—Be a part of the conversation. Take turns listening and speaking. Write down one way you joined in the conversation:

_____

_____

5. Ask questions—Show that you care about what the other person is saying by asking questions. Write down one question you asked:

_____

_____

6. Think about how the conversation went.

What is one thing you did well?

_____

What is one thing you can improve for next time?

_____

Conclusion

You did it! You completed all of the activities in this workbook.

You deserve 1,000 belly rubs, 800 chew toys, and 50 dog treats. Or maybe you have a different idea for a reward, but whatever it is, you've earned it! I hope you feel proud, accomplished, and more equipped to manage your emotions, distress, and interactions.

While you should definitely take a moment to think about your achievement, you should also not make the mistake of thinking you are "done" with DBT! Keep this workbook handy so that you can top up your skills as needed. The more you practice, the more mindful, strong, confident, and connected you will be!

Thank you for joining me on your DBT journey. I hope we can have more adventures together soon!

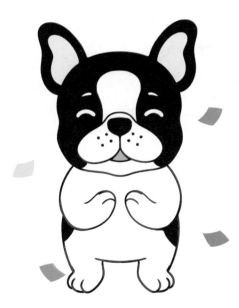

Answers to Activity 29:

I thought you were a snob at first, but you're actually cool. PASSIVE-AGGRESSIVE	I understand your point of view. Can I explain my perspective? ASSERTIVE	Oh great, I get to sit next to you! (When you don't like the person) PASSIVE-AGGRESSIVE
It's nothing. (When something is bothering you) PASSIVE	I'll tell everyone your secret unless you do this for me AGGRESSIVE	I can't help with the project tonight. Can we do it tomorrow? ASSERTIVE
When you blow off our plans, I feel frustrated and unimportant. ASSERTIVE	I'll do whatever you want to do. (When you have a preference) PASSIVE	You aren't going to come with us? You're such a baby! AGGRESSIVE

Note to Parents, Guardians, and Caregivers

Traditional DBT often includes a group for parents and caregivers. Why? Because you play a pivotal role in helping your child to manage their emotions and make wise-mind decisions! Moreover, the skills in this workbook can help you practice wise-mind parenting.

Wise-mind parenting means acting intentionally as opposed to impulsively. It's showing your child empathy while also setting and maintaining clear boundaries. It's validating your child's emotions but also holding them accountable for their behavior. In short, wise-mind parenting creates a nurturing but structured environment where your child can thrive.

While a wise-mind parenting "how to" would require a separate workbook, here are a few tips for helping your child on their DBT journey:

- Set aside time to help your child practice the strategies in this workbook.

- Provide encouragement but refrain from excessive reassurance, rescue, or other forms of protection. Remember that your ultimate goal is for your child to be able to manage their emotions and interactions independently. While it's tempting to step in and "save" your child from difficult situations, this will not help them in the long run.

- Instead, talk through the problem with your child. Help them explore their thoughts and emotions. Ask them which skills might be applicable to the situation. This will ultimately improve your child's self-confidence, as they realize they are capable of working through challenges on their own!

- Remind your child of coping strategies they've successfully used in the past.

- Validate how your child is feeling without trying to "fix" things for them.

- Express confidence in your child's ability to be effective in the situation.

- Celebrate your child's successes, however small they may seem.

- Be willing to seek out professional support, if needed. If your child struggles to implement the skills in this workbook due to the nature or severity of their symptoms, contact a mental health care provider for assessment. While DBT is often an effective treatment for self-harm and suicidality, these symptoms should always be monitored by a licensed professional.

Author Bio

Lindsay Schwartz is a clinical social worker and psychotherapist with over two decades of experience working with children and families. She has served as a consultant to various school districts in addition to maintaining a private therapy practice. Lindsay first taught DBT when she was in graduate school and has been hooked ever since! In her free time, she enjoys reading, writing, and spending time in nature.

FREE BONUS

Join me and dive into the captivating stories of extraordinary sports heroes and fearless entrepreneurs. I can't wait to share their remarkable tales of innovation and determination with you. In addition to the inspiring stories, I have included some fantastic coloring pages that will spark your creativity!

So, what are you waiting for? Claim these free bonuses by scanning the QR code below or typing riccagarden.com/ronny_freebies into your web browser.

(Note: You must be 16 years or older to sign up, so grab your parent for help if you need to.)

Your Frenchie,

RONNY

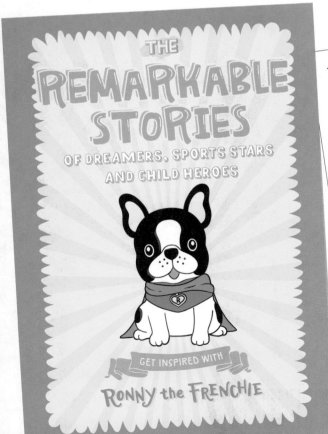

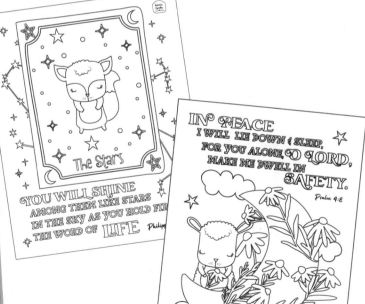

Made in United States
Troutdale, OR
08/12/2025

33575632R10053